THE

CANNABIS OIL

GUIDE

Various Disease Treatments

Using Cannabis Oil

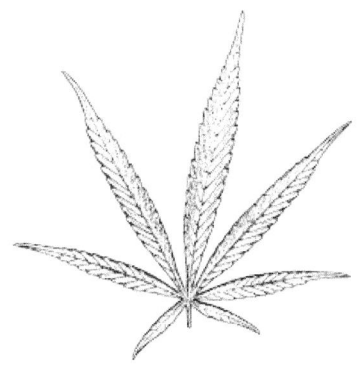

By Martin Pals

Table of content

Introduction

For some time, the medical industry has sought alternatives in the treatment of certain ailments. This is because of the persistence of some health conditions even after some drugs have been taken. A lot of ailments have proven stubborn hence the search for alternative medication.

As technology has evolved, research into the medical world has increased astronomically with the limelight being shown towards the use of natural herbs.

Among such herbs is cannabis oil, which is derived from the Sativa plant. Cannabis is a naturally growing herb that has been used for thousands of years to treat different health conditions. It's also used in making perfumes, soaps, candles, and some other foods and supplements.

Cannabis is a very powerful oil with the ability to treat numerous health conditions, and only small amounts are needed for it to have a powerful effect on the body and mind—hence it is termed a wonder plant. Though serious research is still ongoing, there have been some success stories on the ability of the oil to treat diverse problems.

The Sativa Plant

Cannabis oil can be traced back to the Sativa plant, which is most commonly bred for its potent, sticky glands that are known as trichomes which are a powerful constituent of the oil and which is responsible for its ability in treating many sicknesses. These trichomes are found to contain high amounts of **tetrahydrocannabinol** (generally known as **THC**), which is the cannabinoid most known for its psychoactive properties and therapeutic usefulness.

Due to concerns about the dangers of marijuana abuse in different countries of the world, the sales and movement of this plant were banned for medicinal use in the United States and many other countries in the 1930s and 1940s. Hence it became illegal to be sold or used during this time. It took decades until these plants came to be considered again as compounds of therapeutic value and medical use, though its uses are highly restricted.

The cannabis plant originated in Central Asia, but today it is grown worldwide and considered to be one of the most popular plants. In the United States, it's a controlled substance by government agencies and is classified as a Schedule I agent; this implies that it's a drug with increased potential for abuse hence there is a caution in the sale and use of the drug.

Numerous diseases and infections which include; **anorexia**, **emesis**, **pain**, **anxieties**, **inflammation**, **multiple sclerosis**, **neurodegenerative disorders**, **Asthma**, **epilepsy**, **glaucoma**, **Osteoporosis**, **schizophrenia**, **cardiovascular disorders**, **cancer**, **obesity**, **skin treatment**, and **metabolic syndrome-**related disorders are known to be treated or have the potential to be treated with cannabis oils and other cannabinoid compounds.

Though research and studies into cannabis oil are limited due to strict government guidelines and limitations in accessing it, a growing number of pediatric patients are also seeking symptom relief with cannabis or cannabinoid treatment, and it has been a quick solution to other problems. This book is a product of deep research into the medicinal importance and other benefits of cannabis oil. It is enriched with so many health issues that cannabis oil has been found to cure.

Cannabinoids, which are components of cannabis oil, are a group of a 21-carbon compound containing terpene-phenolic compounds that are produced expressly by cannabis species. These compounds may be referred to as phytocannabinoids.

Although delta-9-tetrahydrocannabinol (the THC) is the primary psychoactive ingredient of the cannabinoids, there are other known compounds with active biologic activity; these compounds include cannabinol, cannabidiol, cannabichromene, cannabigerol, tetrahydrocannabivarin, and popular delta-8-THC.

Cannabidiol is known to have significant pain, stress-relieving, and anti-inflammatory activity even in the absence of the psychoactive effect of delta-9-THC.

How to Obtain and Use Cannabis

Individuals who use cannabis oil as a means of treating different health conditions ingest it into their body with an oral syringe or by adding it to a fluid that masks its potency. The dose measurement and frequency are mainly based on the health condition being treated and the patient's cannabis tolerance level; this level can be ascertained through a doctor or health expert. Most patients often start with a small amount and then increase the treatment doses over a long period depending on their cannabis tolerance level. You need to know your level of tolerance to avoid abusing this drug.

It's difficult if not impossible to buy cannabis oil online or at a local pharmaceutical store, the reason is not far-fetched as there are huge regulations on the sales of the oil. Some states provide individuals with cannabis strictly for medical conditions, and this may require a medical note or proof of injury and illness from a hospital to qualify to access this drug. Also, to access it, you can also join a collective health group, which is a group of patients who grow and share medical cannabis with a legal right to do so. If you are to use cannabis oil, make sure it's purchased from a reputable company that has the legal right to sell pure and lab-tested oils to people.

Fake cannabis oils online

There are many fake cannabis oils online, and most of them are imported and sold to patients who are in dire need of this oil. This is why it is good to read books and ask questions before paying for any cannabis oil.

Some of the cannabis which is seen online is adulterated and wrongly produced and should not be used in treating any health problem. Medical experts recommend that you go through the legal and safe means of obtaining cannabis oil to ensure its health benefits and avoid any possible side effects.

As a word of caution, please do not use cannabis oil, or any cannabis product, or any cannabidiol drug if you are pregnant or could become pregnant within a short time!

There is some available evidence which suggests that women who use cannabis oil or products during the time of conception or while pregnant may increase the risk of their child being born with possible birth defects or at a very low weight, also breastfeeding mothers are advised not to use this drug.

Cannabis Oil

Cannabis is a very powerful medicinal herb with a very long history of curing many health problems and skin infections. According to medical history accrued over the years, cannabis has been cultivated in various regions of the world for millennia, and its cultivation has grown with time as a result of its frequent demand and medical purpose.

Cannabis, which is also known as **marijuana**, refers to the liquids or oil derived from the **Cannabis Sativa plant**, which is typically cultivated for their potent trichomes and other important usages. These seemingly sticky glands contain high amounts of a substance which is referred to as THC or tetrahydrocannabinol, a substance known for its psychotropic abilities and cancer curing capacity.

Cannabis oil is found to be a strong and sticky resinous substance that is derived from the cannabis plant and which has found to be of great importance in the medical world. This oil has become very popular and infamous in recent years due to the movement for legalized marijuana in some countries as opposed to the laws imposed on its transportation from different parts of the world. Found to possess CBD and THC, there are a good number of health benefits that users of cannabis oil derive from it.

It is deduced from the resin of the cannabis flowers. Due to the increasing number of health issues that cannabis oil has been found to solve, it is becoming a clarion call for all to take advantage of the numerous uses of this herb. This book is written so that the reader will gain useful insights on how to use cannabis oil in solving those problems that the use of chemical drugs has been unable to solve.

Cannabis is being transported to different countries and has found usefulness, though largely misused. It has different names, according to drugs.com. Cannabis is also known as Ganja, Grass, Hashish, Hemp, Indian hemp, marijuana, Pot, reefer, weed, and lots of different names given to it in various countries of the world.

Extracting the Cannabis Oil

To extract cannabis oil from the Sativa plant, a solvent extraction process is used during this process, which returns roughly 3-5 grams of oil per ounce of flower product that is used during the extraction. You can also use grain alcohol or isopropyl alcohol as a solvent during the extraction process, and you will then strain the result of the mixture, which will leave cannabis oil as the residue.

This process is a rather involved and lengthy process that requires the use of some equipment to achieve, and in countries where cannabis is legal, there are many places to access high-quality cannabis oil that has already been extracted. It is my prediction that though the cannabis leaf is widely misused, in the long term this oil will be a breakthrough in the medical world as enough research is currently ongoing on the usefulness of this oil. This oil is also seen to be a very good skin nourishing oil, and one is forced to ask why this important oil with such medical uses is so strictly limited and restricted.

The importance of Cannabis Oil

The medical importance of this oil cannot be over-emphasized. Cannabis oil has a wide range of effects on human health, and it has been linked to a diverse number of health challenges and issues, ranging from migraines and stress to lack of appetite and low sex drive in humans.

Cannabis oil has even been connected to reducing the risk of certain cancers even more than chemical drugs can do, as well as reduce body pains. It is also known to help in strengthening the heart and helping people get a good night's sleep after a very stressful day or after strenuous activities.

There are some ways to use cannabis oil in solving many health problems, depending on what you want relief from; it can be useful in treating virtually any issues as well as in treating some known skin infections.

Medical Research into cannabis essential oil is highly regulated, and science is still in the early stages of its development and uses of the oil. It is the hope of science that in the nearest future, as technology is evolving in the medical direction that more research will be conducted and that the regulatory bodies restricting the use of cannabis oil will become more welcoming to its potential to treat people safely without any side effects or complications.

Therefore let's look at the health benefits of using cannabis oil.

1. Stress and Anxiety

Stress, anxiety, and other related emotional disorders are an increasing modern concern that is fast spreading and has a strong base in the United States. The medical world is continuously looking at numerous potential and natural alternatives in resolving emotional disorders. There have been many highly ineffective and dangerous prescriptions used to treat these disorders, and there is a need for an alternative. On average, **almost 6 in every 10 Americans** suffer from stress and anxiety on a daily basis, while they have traditionally relied on drugs to get over this stress, the high increase of this disorder is a sure proof that a better alternative is needed in solving this problem.

Cannabis oil is, therefore, worth exploring and studying further as it can relax the troubled mind and stimulate the release of pleasure hormones in the bodies of those that use it. This combination of effects can lead to speedy stress reduction and provide a way for feelings of calmness and general well being of the entire body. As has been pointed out in the sections above, cannabis oil can help in getting a sound night's sleep/rest which is known to reduce anxiety and stress.

Cannabinoids which are found in the oil are responsible for creating a positive emotional response in the body's nervous system as it helps to relax the entire system and prepare the body for work later on. Several recent studies have demonstrated the potential value of cannabis oil in stress relief as well as solving other related issues like insomnia.

One recent study that reveals this is an Israeli study which was published in 2013, which demonstrated that treating the body with cannabinoids following some form of traumatic experience might help to reduce and control the emotional responses to that traumatic event and prevent stress-related responses gotten as a result of a traumatic experience.

Researchers also discovered that cannabinoids were effective in reducing stress receptors in the body's hippocampus, which is the area of the brain responsible for emotional response and control of trauma.

Also, cannabis treatments were found to be very effective in reducing anxiety and restlessness in military veterans who are suffering from PTSD. Whether cannabis oil is inhaled or orally administered, it leads to a wide range of positive nervous system effects that include an increased feeling of body pleasure and calmness. While there is a need for further research on how cannabis oil can help in stress relief, the research conducted so far as well as a large body of anecdotal evidence found has been very promising for the future use of cannabis oil to treat anxiety, stress, and sleeping disorders. The natural compounds found in cannabis oil like THC, which gives the cannabis a drug classification, are very good for the release of the pleasure homes as has been discussed above.

Also for people who suffer from insomnia and constant anxiety during the nighttime hours or those who always struggle to get a sound, restful night of undisturbed sleep, you need to worry no more as cannabis oil works like a charm in getting you to easily fall asleep and sustaining you throughout the whole night's sleep. By relaxing your body, mind, and by inducing a lower energy level in your body, it will be easier to get your heartbeat rate down and clear your head to prepare you for a long night of peaceful slumber without any of the body aches or anxiety that you might have experienced before.

2. Appetite and Obesity

Cannabis has a well-known history of its ability to increase an individual's appetite for food. It is also possible that it has potential to be a good supplement for people who need to increase their weight as a result of a sickness that made them lose a lot of weight or because of an eating disorder like anorexia nervosa that can induce a weight loss in the body.

Cannabis oil can serve as a stimulant to the body's digestive system and induce hunger in those lacking the appetite to eat. While cannabis oil can induce taste for food by helping release hormones responsible for hunger, it is important that some certain hormones responsible for hunger suppression can also be stimulated by cannabinoids which are found in cannabis oil.

In summary, depending on which hormone gets stimulated in the long run, cannabis oil might also be very effective in reducing appetite and controlling obesity in the body of those its users. To effectively control obesity, it is important to manipulate the cannabinoids in cannabis oil to stimulate the appropriate hormones for any purpose in which it is used to achieve.

Cannabis oil may be very much effective in treating both obesity and eating disorders like anorexia simultaneously in the nearest future. Therefore those who wish to reduce weight can take refuge in cannabis oil to achieve a quick result. If you have been looking for an appetite booster, look no more.

3. Asthma

Asthma is a general respiratory disease that affects up to 300 million people around the world. Asthma is responsible for numerous deaths every year, and the search for a natural and effective treatment to curtail the growth and propagation of this ailment has been ongoing for many years and will remain at the forefront of research in the medical world.

So the million-dollar question is how cannabis oil can help in the treatment of Asthma.

Cannabis has been traditionally used to treat asthma for many years in Chinese and Indian medicine. With such capabilities, cannabis oil may be an effective natural treatment for asthmatic patients because of its natural anti-inflammatory ability and its ability to dilate the bronchial tubes, which are a pathway for in the inflow of oxygen into the respiratory system.

It should be known that during the early 1970s there were several research studies which investigated the bronchodilatory effects of cannabis for people suffering from asthma and most of this research was positive—hence, it can be said to be a good drug for treating Asthma. While there is little available evidence regarding the use of cannabis oil for asthmatics it has been found to improve the symptoms of Asthma and hence could be used in its treatment and cure. Also, early reports have revealed the presence of an active ingredient in cannabis essential oil that can prevent the effects of Asthma.

4. Heart Health

As cannabis oil continues to be a good alternative for the treatment of many physical problems, the heart is not left out. This is because cannabis oil contains active antioxidant properties that have proven to be very beneficial for the total wellbeing and functioning of the heart. Animal studies conducted to this effect have demonstrated that treatment with cannabis oil can prevent numerous cardiovascular diseases most of which include: atherosclerosis, heart attacks, catarrh, and strokes.

This animal study finds application to human heart conditions; this is because the cannabinoids could cause the blood vessels to relax further and dilate creating the pathway to improved blood and air circulation and also reduced blood pressure within the heart. This study is a breakthrough, and other forthcoming studies will further prove that cannabis oil has major implications for the health of the heart.

This study also reveals that those who regularly consume cannabis oil have a reduced chance of having a stroke. The increasing number of stroke is drawing a global concern, so anything that can prevent it especially important to know.

5. Pain Relief

One of the popular historical applications of the cannabis plant oil has been to ease pains and inflammation in the body.

There is evidence that cannabis oil has been used for thousands of years to resolve these purposes. Also, there is corresponding modern evidence that shows cannabis and cannabis oil is effective in relieving body pain and inflammation by inhibiting the neural transmission in the body's pain pathways such that the neural transmission does not get to go deep into the body. The cannabis oil has the potential to cure chronic pain as well as inflammation, which is why many cancer patients all over the world choose to take it while undergoing chemotherapy and medical experts have highly recommended it.

Many people often take cannabis oil to deal with severe rheumatism and arthritis as well as other chronic pains found in the body especially among the older ones. Other recent research has demonstrated that it can be used to alleviate neuropathic pain in most patients. It is considered to be very safe when taken in appropriate prescriptions, and studies have found that it is largely well tolerated, unlike the leaf which is widely misused by many.

6. Cancer

There has been a considerable amount of excitement in the medical world regarding the ability of cannabis oil to cure cancer. This great news often makes headlines or published in most medical journals. Unfortunately, these headlines are often overly optimistic and can be misleading for both patients and their families who do not truly understand the truth of what cannabis oil can do and the things it cannot do to cancer patients.

First of all, it should be clearly stated out that the large majority of scientific research into the effects of cannabis oil in treating cancer had been conducted either on animals or in the laboratory. The implication is that we need to exercise a degree of caution in extrapolating the results to human subjects; however, the fact that the results gotten so far reveals it can cure cancer in a human. If any drug for treating the cancerous cells is discovered, it is first tried with animals to check the effect before using it on humans. This is achieved by injecting cancerous cells in the body of the animal, which in most cases a rat is used since it is a mammal. Then the cancer cells are allowed to get hold of the animal before the potential treatment is injected and watched to observe the effect of it in treating the disease.

In light of this testimony, scientists have been able to discover that many different cannabinoids in the cannabis plant have a range of positive effects under laboratory conditions in treating cancer.

These positive effects include:

• Triggering the immediate death of the cancer cells, this process is commonly known as apoptosis.

• Preventing and reducing the division of cancerous cells.

• Preventing new blood vessels from becoming tumors which lead to the formation of cancer in the body of the victim.

• Reducing the risk and rate of cancerous cells from spreading throughout the body and attacking the healthy neighboring tissue.

It should be known that up to now the most positive effects results have been seen when using a combination of purified THC in combination with cannabidiol. This is a cannabinoid that counteracts the psychoactive effect of THC, and a more positive result is observed on a daily basis.

Other medical research has revealed that cannabis oil is highly effective when used in combination with other chemotherapy medications in treating cancer. Although there is no hard and fast evidence that cannabis oil is a miracle cure-all for cancer treatment, the early signs are very glaring, and further research into it will soon help us find the answers that the world is earnestly waiting for.

As has been pointed out in this paragraph, the combination of cannabis oil and other chemotherapy has proven to be useful in treating cancer. This is one of the recent improvements in the medical world as so many people suffer from cancer and any treatment of this is a quantum leap.

Another treatment of cancer, which is gaining more attention in the health industry, is the use of nano-technology, though for now, it is still the product of laboratory investigation. Treating with cannabis oil remains the safest for now since it has no side effect and it has proven to be successful.

When treating cancer, the suggestion is always to take three doses of cannabis oil each day, and subsequently, increase the amount of the dose until 1 gram per day is consumed on daily. A full treatment of cancer is believed to take 90 days if the patient follows the prescriptions. It should be known that the sale of cannabis oil is still illegal in many countries though it can be gotten in the United States. The process of getting it has been explained above. Though due to the significant amount of research being done on its medical applications and usage, and some reputable sources and agencies have put out guides for the access and use of cannabis oil for the treatment of the cancer disease. Hence this oil can be sought with permission and may not be allowed to be imported from other countries, especially from countries where its use is illegal. Thus, when searching online for this oil, you must be very observant to avoid being scammed by fake online dealers.

7. Skin Protection

Cannabis oil can be used topically to maintain healthy and glowing skin. When applied topically on the skin, cannabis oil can help stimulate the shedding of older and dead skin cells, exfoliation of the skin, and promote the growth of new skin cells to replace the older ones. Applying cannabis oil, as well as aloe after-sun gel, witch hazel, tea tree oil or other aloe-based lotion after shaving can help the skin feel cool, relaxed, comfortable, and may help keep it smooth later. You may also try using radiant skin silk body lotion or other lotion recommended by a dermatologist, which has calming calendula, chamomile, and sunflower oil on your skin as it will help retain your skin color. But the cannabis is a good treatment for the skin even for razor bumps.

Cannabinoids can aid to enhance the production of lipids, which help fight chronic skin conditions including razor bumps, acne, and psoriasis. There is a possibility that cannabis oil can help prevent the signs of aging like wrinkles, skin spots, blemishes. And other body aging signs on the body because it is high in natural antioxidants that help fight against cellular damage caused by free radicals and help to nourish the skin to be smooth and ever glowing. One of the most powerful uses of cannabis is in the protection of the skin. To achieve this, cannabis oil can be consumed or applied externally on the skin as it has been most effective. By reducing the effect and amount of stress that we feel inside the body, cannabis oil can also be very helpful in preventing skin diseases that tend to break out during times of anxiety and stress like eczema or rosacea.

This is the reason while the global demand for cannabis oil is growing astronomically because of the need to maintain the skin color and beauty.

8. Eye Health

There is available evidence which demonstrates the ability and usefulness of cannabis oil to treat some eye conditions like glaucoma and macular degeneration, which is common among many people. Glaucoma is a serious optic nerve disease of the eye that might lead to loss of proper vision and even total blindness when not properly managed or treated.

Glaucoma is caused by the accumulation of fluid within the eye, which results in too much pressure on the retina, lens, and optic nerve of the eyes. While numerous factors may contribute to nerve damage in many people suffering from glaucoma, it is completely related and linked to intraocular pressure or IOP.

The American Glaucoma Society has confirmed the place of cannabis oil in treating this eye problem. The society reveals that cannabis oil can reduce the level of IOP in both those suffering from glaucoma and the potential glaucoma patients. Unfortunately, its effects in solving the IOP level on the eyes are temporary, and patients would need to use cannabis oil only for few hours to shore up the effects as we expect more research on its ability to completely cure the eye problem.

9. For Treating Seizures

Though there has been some controversy over this, there is still some evidence emanating from small-scale studies carried out using cannabis oil. This anecdotal report suggests that the cannabidiol content of cannabis oil can be very useful in preventing seizures and could be used as a novel treatment for epilepsy in humans.

Though the truth is that there is not enough evidence to back up its use in treating seizures and the limited evidence that is available so far has proven contradictory among some scientists. Among the seizure patients who were treated with cannabis oil, it should be noted that of none of them experienced any adverse side effects as a result of the treatment and that more studies in future may prove to be very useful in treating this problem.

10. Other Potential Benefits of the Cannabis oil

Headaches and Migraines:

It has been proven that cannabis oil is an effective tool in the treatment of migraines and headache. When the oil is topically applied at the temples or the spot of intensity for a migraine or a headache, it is found to be an effective way to get relief. As a result of this, many people obtain prescriptions for cannabis and cannabis oil due to its potent defense against crippling headaches and other body pain. Hence it is very useful for getting quick relief when having a headache.

The United States' laws on the Cannabis Oil

The use and sale of cannabis and cannabis oil for medicinal purposes are now legalized in 25 states in the United States though you shouldn't expect to be able to walk into a shop and buy it as you may not see it sold in public stores or pharmacists. To have access to this product, you may require a medical certificate and a proof of illness to acquire cannabis oil from the state, but you can obtain this proof easily, and you will be given access to it.

To have quick access to this product, you may have to join a collective group, i.e., a group of patients that share and sometimes grow medicinal cannabis due to their health problems. This method remains the fastest means of getting access to cannabis oil. Or you can further contact me on how to go about getting this in oil.

You need to be aware that there are numerous scams and fake dealers online promising to sell medicinal cannabis to you. These persons only aim at deceiving you and getting away with your money. Hence it is very important that you do your research and find a well-known dealer well before you go ahead with your purchase. Experts' advise that you purchase only oil produced by a reputable company who test the product in a lab, so you don't have complications or don't find yourself deceived into using fake cannabis in treating your problems.

The Difference between the Cannabis oil and Hemp oil

Often, many people confuse the two without having proper knowledge of what the difference between the two herbs. It is pertinent to know that both cannabis and hemp oil are derived from the same species, the "Cannabis sativa." Unlike cannabis oil, hemp oil is quite different due to its production. Therefore, hemp is a high growing species of the plant Sativa, which is commonly produced for industrial purposes like topical ointments, fiber, paper, and other industrial purposes.

Unlike cannabis oil, hemp oil has only trace amounts of THC (in little quantity) and hence is not considered to have the same medicinal value as that of cannabis oil. It is also important to know that both hemp oil and cannabis oil also contain the cannabidiol or CBD, which contain medicinal properties, notwithstanding, cannabis oil is of good medicinal value as compared to hemp oil. However, it is found that there is far less of this compound (THC) contained in hemp than cannabis oil, hence the superiority of cannabis oil over hemp in solving medical issues. According to results of the recent study, cannabis oil is actually around 100 times more potent than hemp oil; this implies that the dose of hemp oil necessary to have an equivalent medicinal effect would be extremely high and less cost effective. This research further speaks of the need for the use of cannabis oil over hemp for a quick result in any health-related issue.

Word of Caution

Although this list clearly outlines that cannabis oil can be an effective remedy for treating many common health conditions, it should be remembered that it is still a potent chemical substance extracted from a plant with high psychotropic substances and hence caution should be taken. Therefore, users should always be very careful in the way and manner cannabis oil is used, this includes the conditions under which the oil is taken. It is advisable that you speak to a professional about combining the oil and present medications before adding any new elements to your health regimen to avoid any complications that may result from the chemical reactions. Also, the use of cannabis oil is restricted/banned by many countries, so it is necessary that you consult local health specialists before you use cannabis oil.

Conclusion

Cannabis is a plant genus which is of three different species: Indica, Sativa, and Ruderalis, and it's been used for both health and medicinal purposes for thousands of years and is still a current trend in the medical world. Cannabis oil has been used in the treatment of many diseases without any side effects or complications. I have to accept the fact that a mild addiction to cannabis is possible, but medical researchers agree that the therapeutic effects of cannabinoids are considerable and should not be ignored. In particular, uses for cannabis oil cannot be stopped or neglected since it has numerous advantages than disadvantages. There is also a method of checking an individual's cannabis tolerance level which makes the use of the oil to be moderated and not be abused.

Smoking marijuana leaf is well known to increase appetite in a person, but the cannabis essential oil can also help to stimulate your digestive system and induce hunger. This ability of cannabis oil is useful for people who are trying to gain weight, especially after an illness or injury which led to the loss of body weight. Cannabis leaf and cannabis oil have also been linked to the prevention of macular degeneration and the treatment of glaucoma especially among the aged persons in the society. As one grows older, cannabis oil is useful in ensuring the total wellbeing of the body. It can keep an individual safe from diseases which is associated with old age. Although research is still ongoing, cannabis oil is considered an option in the treatment and prevention of cancer as the available research has suggested. Using cannabis oil in cancer prevention or treatment may help reduce tumor size and alleviate possible weakness, pain, nausea, and a lack of appetite in a cancer patient. Cannabis oil may improve the health of cancer patients by triggering cancer cell death and cutting off the pathway of the blood supply to the tumor. Other case reports into the cancer treatment have found that cannabis oil is a non-toxic chemotherapy alternative that has the ability to increase vitality in patients with acute lymphoblastic leukemia.

Aside its usefulness in treating to diseases, Cannabinoids found in cannabis produce lipids, which can help treat dry skin, dandruff or acne, and help to improve the skin's appearance. The oil is also seen to fight any free-radical damage on the skin and reduce the stress linked with eczema, rosacea, and acne. In fact, cannabis oil is generally used for the total skin treatment; there are also cannabis oil benefits for the hair. Veterinary studies on animals have revealed that cannabis may prevent heart conditions such as heart attacks, atherosclerosis, stroke, hypertension, and coronary heart disease, which is also applicable to the human. Post-traumatic stress disorder (PTSD) is a common psychiatric condition that results from life-threatening experiences such as military wars or combats, serious accidents, or natural disasters, and emotional trauma. From the above, it is very visible to the blind and audible to the deaf that cannabis oil is very important if anyone must live a healthy life.

www.ingramcontent.com/pod-product-compliance
Lightning Source LLC
Chambersburg PA
CBHW072009230526
45468CB00020B/1084